Younger for Life in 30 days Cookbook

30 days of healthy meals that can make you feel great and look your best. New, science-backed recipes for autophagy can help you rejuvenate your body and mind.

Maria W. Irvin

Table of Contents

Embrace the Fountain of Youth: Introduction to Younger for Life

Imagine... waking up with skin that radiates, energy that bounds, and a zest for life that whispers "youthful." We often romanticize the fountain of youth, a mythical spring promising to reverse the clock. But what if I told you this magic potion wasn't hidden in a forbidden forest, but nestled right on your plate?

Welcome to Younger for Life, your 30-day guide to unlocking the fountain's secret: Autojuvenation food. Forget fad diets and quick fixes. This revolution is about harnessing the power of delicious, everyday ingredients to awaken your body's innate ability to renew.

Let's face it, aging isn't always graceful. Wrinkles creep in, energy dwindles, and that youthful spark sometimes feels like a flicker. But these changes aren't inevitable sentences from the aging gods. They're largely the result of four pesky horsemen: oxidative damage, inflammation, glycation, and stress. These villains wage a silent war on our cells, stealing away vitality and leaving us feeling older than our years.

But fear not, noble knight! Younger for Life serves up your armor and weapons – a culinary arsenal packed with vibrant, flavor-bursting dishes specifically designed to combat these villains and reignite your inner fire. Forget bland, restrictive regimes. Here, you'll find recipes that tantalize your taste buds while unleashing the autojuvenation powerhouses within. Think juicy berry smoothies fighting free radicals, turmeric-infused salmon extinguishing inflammation, and dark chocolate peanut butter bars melting stress away.

This 30-day journey isn't just about the food, though. It's about a holistic approach to reclaiming your youthful vibrancy. We'll explore the science behind autojuvenation, delve into complementary practices like mindful eating and exercise, and even discover simple skincare and sleep hacks to enhance your glow.

So, are you ready to shed the chains of aging and embrace the fountain within? Crack open this book, arm yourself with your fork, and prepare to embark on a delicious adventure. It's time to say goodbye to tired, hello to thriving!

This introduction aims to be engaging, informative, and motivating. It sets the stage for the 30-day journey and establishes the core concepts of autojuvenation food and holistic living. You can adjust the tone and specific examples to reflect your unique writing style and the overall brand of your cookbook.

I hope this helps you kickstart your introduction!

The Four Horsemen of Aging and How to Defeat Them: A Culinary Approach"

As we navigate the journey of aging, it's crucial to understand and combat the four horsemen that contribute to the aging process: Oxidative Damage, Inflammation, Glycation, and Stress. In this culinary guide, we'll explore the impact of each horseman and discover delicious recipes designed to fortify your body against these aging factors.

1. Oxidative Damage: Foods to Fight Free Radicals and Boost Antioxidants

Description: Oxidative damage occurs when free radicals attack healthy cells, leading to aging. Combat this process by incorporating foods rich in antioxidants into your diet.

Recipes:

1. Berry Blast Smoothie:

   - Ingredients: Mixed berries, spinach, Greek yogurt, chia seeds, almond milk.
   - Instructions: Blend ingredients until smooth, creating a refreshing antioxidant-packed smoothie.

2. Turmeric Salmon with Roasted Vegetables:

- Ingredients: Salmon fillet, turmeric, olive oil, mixed vegetables.
- Instructions: Marinate salmon with turmeric, roast alongside colorful vegetables for a powerful anti-oxidative dish.

2. Inflammation: Calming the Fire Within with Anti-Inflammatory Foods

Description: Chronic inflammation accelerates aging. Choose foods that possess anti-inflammatory properties to keep the flames at bay.

Recipes:

1. Mediterranean Quinoa Salad:

- Ingredients: Quinoa, cherry tomatoes, cucumber, feta cheese, olives, olive oil.
- Instructions: Toss ingredients together to create a vibrant salad with anti-inflammatory benefits.

2. Spicy Chicken Curry with Coconut Milk:

- Ingredients: Chicken, curry spices, coconut milk, vegetables.
- Instructions: Simmer ingredients to perfection, creating a flavorful curry that fights inflammation.

3. Glycation: Sweeten Your Life Without Sacrificing Youth

- Description: Glycation occurs when sugar molecules attach to proteins, contributing to aging. Choose wisely by opting for naturally sweetened recipes.

Recipes:

1. Chia Seed Pudding with Berries:

- Ingredients: Chia seeds, almond milk, berries, honey.
- Instructions: Mix ingredients and refrigerate overnight for a delectable, youth-preserving pudding.

2. Grilled Salmon with Herbs and Lemon:

- Ingredients: Salmon fillet, fresh herbs, lemon, olive oil.
- Instructions: Grill salmon with herbs and a squeeze of lemon for a naturally sweetened dish.

4. Stress: Nourishing Your Mind and Body to Combat Stress Aging

- Description: Chronic stress contributes significantly to the aging process. Nourish your body with stress-relieving foods to maintain a youthful balance.

- Recipes:

1. Chamomile Tea with Honey and Lavender:

- Ingredients: Chamomile tea, honey, dried lavender.
- Instructions: Brew tea, add honey and lavender for a soothing beverage that calms both mind and body.

2. Dark Chocolate Peanut Butter Bars:

- Ingredients: Dark chocolate, peanut butter, oats, honey.
- Instructions: Create no-bake bars combining the goodness of dark chocolate and the stress-relieving properties of peanut butter.

By incorporating these recipes into your culinary repertoire, you embark on a journey to defy the four horsemen of aging. Embrace the power of antioxidants, anti-inflammatory ingredients, natural sweeteners, and stress-relieving foods to savor a life of vitality and youthfulness.

30 Days of Autojuvenation Meals: Ignite Your Inner Fountain of Youth

Week 1: Revitalize

Day 1: Berry Bliss Smoothie Bowl with Chia Seeds and Hemp Hearts

Ingredients:

- 1 cup mixed berries (strawberries, blueberries, raspberries)
- 1 banana
- 1/2 cup Greek yogurt
- 2 tablespoons chia seeds
- 1 tablespoon hemp hearts
- 1/2 cup almond milk

Instructions:

1. Blend berries, banana, Greek yogurt, chia seeds, hemp hearts, and almond milk until smooth.
2. Pour into a bowl and top with additional berries, chia seeds, and hemp hearts.

Day 2: Sunrise Scramble with Spinach, Tomatoes, and Avocado

Ingredients:

- 2 eggs
- 1 cup fresh spinach
- 1/2 cup cherry tomatoes, halved
- 1/2 avocado, sliced
- Salt and pepper to taste

Instructions:

1. In a pan, scramble eggs over medium heat.
2. Add spinach and cook until wilted.
3. Stir in cherry tomatoes and cook until heated through.
4. Serve with sliced avocado on top. Season with salt and pepper.

Day 3: Lentil Soup with Kale and Lemon Garlic Zest

Ingredients:

- 1 cup dried lentils, rinsed
- 1 onion, diced
- 2 carrots, chopped
- 2 celery stalks, chopped
- 3 cloves garlic, minced
- 4 cups vegetable broth
- 2 cups kale, chopped
- Zest of 1 lemon
- Salt and pepper to taste

Instructions:

1. In a large pot, sauté onion, carrots, celery, and garlic until softened.
2. Add lentils and vegetable broth. Bring to a boil, then simmer until lentils are tender.
3. Stir in kale, lemon zest, salt, and pepper. Cook until kale is wilted.

Day 4: Salmon with Roasted Asparagus and Turmeric Tahini Sauce

Ingredients:

- 2 salmon fillets
- 1 bunch asparagus, trimmed
- 2 tablespoons olive oil
- 1 teaspoon turmeric
- Salt and pepper to taste
- Tahini sauce for drizzling

Instructions:

1. Preheat oven to 400°F (200°C).
2. Place salmon and asparagus on a baking sheet.
3. Drizzle with olive oil, sprinkle with turmeric, salt, and pepper.
4. Roast in the oven for 15-20 minutes.
5. Serve with a drizzle of tahini sauce.

Day 5: Spicy Black Bean Burger on Sprouted Grain Bun with Mango Salsa

Ingredients:

- 2 black bean burger patties (store-bought or homemade)
- 2 sprouted grain buns
- 1 cup mango, diced
- 1/4 cup red onion, finely chopped
- 1 jalapeño, seeded and minced
- Fresh cilantro, chopped

Instructions:

1. Cook black bean burgers according to package or recipe instructions.
2. In a bowl, mix mango, red onion, jalapeño, and cilantro to make salsa.
3. Place burgers on sprouted grain buns and top with mango salsa.

Day 6: Rainbow Veggie Stir-Fry with Quinoa and Cashews

Ingredients:

- 1 cup quinoa, cooked
- 1 tablespoon sesame oil
- 1 bell pepper, sliced
- 1 carrot, julienned
- 1 zucchini, sliced
- 1 cup broccoli florets
- 1/4 cup soy sauce
- 2 tablespoons rice vinegar

- 1 tablespoon maple syrup
- 1/2 cup cashews, toasted

Instructions:

1. Heat sesame oil in a pan. Stir-fry bell pepper, carrot, zucchini, and broccoli until tender-crisp.
2. In a small bowl, mix soy sauce, rice vinegar, and maple syrup. Pour over vegetables.
3. Stir in cooked quinoa and toss until well combined.
4. Top with toasted cashews before serving.

Day 7: Coconut Curry Chicken with Sweet Potato Noodles

Ingredients:

- 2 boneless, skinless chicken breasts, thinly sliced
- 2 sweet potatoes, spiralized into noodles
- 1 can (14 oz) coconut milk
- 2 tablespoons red curry paste
- 1 tablespoon fish sauce
- 1 tablespoon lime juice
- Fresh cilantro for garnish

Instructions:

1. In a pan, cook chicken slices until browned.
2. Add coconut milk, red curry paste, fish sauce, and lime juice. Simmer until chicken is cooked through.
3. In a separate pan, sauté sweet potato noodles until tender.

4. Serve curry over sweet potato noodles, garnished with fresh cilantro.

Week 2: Build Your Foundation

Day 8: Detox Salad with Grilled Halloumi and Lemon Herb Vinaigrette

Ingredients:

- 4 cups mixed greens (spinach, arugula, kale)
- 1 cup cherry tomatoes, halved
- 1 cucumber, sliced
- 1/2 cup red onion, thinly sliced
- 200g halloumi cheese, grilled and sliced
- 1/4 cup olive oil
- 2 tablespoons lemon juice
- 1 teaspoon Dijon mustard
- 1 tablespoon fresh herbs (parsley, mint), chopped
- Salt and pepper to taste

Instructions:

1. In a large bowl, combine mixed greens, cherry tomatoes, cucumber, and red onion.
2. Top with grilled halloumi slices.
3. In a small bowl, whisk together olive oil, lemon juice, Dijon mustard, fresh herbs, salt, and pepper.
4. Drizzle the vinaigrette over the salad before serving.

Day 9: Watermelon Gazpacho with Mint and Toasted Almonds

Ingredients:

- 4 cups watermelon, diced
- 1 cucumber, peeled and diced
- 1 bell pepper, diced
- 1/4 cup red onion, finely chopped
- 2 tablespoons fresh mint, chopped
- 2 tablespoons red wine vinegar
- 2 tablespoons olive oil
- Salt and pepper to taste
- 1/4 cup almonds, toasted and chopped

Instructions:

1. In a blender, combine watermelon, cucumber, bell pepper, red onion, mint, red wine vinegar, and olive oil.
2. Blend until smooth. Season with salt and pepper.
3. Chill in the refrigerator before serving.
4. Garnish with toasted almonds just before serving.

Day 10: Quinoa Tabouli with Fresh Herbs and Cucumber

Ingredients:

- 1 cup quinoa, cooked and cooled
- 1 cucumber, diced
- 1 cup cherry tomatoes, halved
- 1/2 cup red onion, finely chopped
- 1/2 cup fresh parsley, chopped
- 1/4 cup fresh mint, chopped
- 2 tablespoons olive oil

- 2 tablespoons lemon juice
- Salt and pepper to taste

Instructions:

1. In a large bowl, combine cooked quinoa, cucumber, cherry tomatoes, red onion, parsley, and mint.
2. In a small bowl, whisk together olive oil, lemon juice, salt, and pepper.
3. Drizzle the dressing over the quinoa mixture and toss until well combined.

Day 11: Green Goddess Smoothie with Almond Milk and Spirulina

Ingredients:

- 1 cup almond milk
- 1 banana
- 1/2 avocado
- Handful of spinach
- 1 tablespoon spirulina powder
- Ice cubes (optional)

Instructions:

1. In a blender, combine almond milk, banana, avocado, spinach, and spirulina.
2. Blend until smooth. Add ice cubes if desired.

Day 12: Whole Wheat Pancakes with Berries and Coconut Yogurt

Ingredients:

- 1 cup whole wheat flour
- 1 tablespoon baking powder
- 1/2 teaspoon cinnamon
- 1 cup almond milk
- 1 tablespoon maple syrup
- 1 teaspoon vanilla extract
- Mixed berries for topping
- Coconut yogurt for topping

Instructions:

1. In a bowl, whisk together whole wheat flour, baking powder, and cinnamon.
2. Add almond milk, maple syrup, and vanilla extract. Mix until just combined.
3. Heat a griddle or non-stick pan. Pour batter onto the hot surface to form pancakes.
4. Cook until bubbles form on the surface, then flip and cook the other side.
5. Top with mixed berries and coconut yogurt.

Day 13: Turkey Meatloaf with Mushroom Gravy and Roasted Brussels Sprouts

Ingredients:

- 1 lb ground turkey
- 1/2 cup breadcrumbs
- 1 egg
- 1/2 cup onion, finely chopped

- 1/4 cup carrot, grated
- 1/4 cup celery, finely chopped
- 2 cloves garlic, minced
- Salt and pepper to taste
- 1 cup mushrooms, sliced
- 1 cup beef or vegetable broth
- 1 tablespoon flour
- Brussels sprouts, halved

Instructions:

1. Preheat the oven to 375°F (190°C).
2. In a bowl, mix ground turkey, breadcrumbs, egg, onion, carrot, celery, garlic, salt, and pepper.
3. Form the mixture into a loaf shape and place it on a baking sheet.
4. Bake for about 45 minutes or until cooked through.
5. Meanwhile, sauté mushrooms in a pan until browned.
6. Sprinkle flour over the mushrooms, stirring to combine.
7. Gradually add broth, stirring until the gravy thickens.
8. Roast Brussels sprouts in the oven until golden.
9. Serve turkey meatloaf with mushroom gravy and roasted Brussels sprouts.

Day 14: Mediterranean Tuna Salad with Whole Wheat Pita Bread

Ingredients:

- 2 cans (5 oz each) tuna, drained
- 1 cup cherry tomatoes, halved
- 1 cucumber, diced
- 1/4 cup red onion, finely chopped
- 1/4 cup Kalamata olives, sliced
- 2 tablespoons feta cheese, crumbled
- 2 tablespoons olive oil
- 1 tablespoon balsamic vinegar
- Salt and pepper to taste
- Whole wheat pita bread

Instructions:

1. In a bowl, combine tuna, cherry tomatoes, cucumber, red onion, olives, and feta.
2. In a small bowl, whisk together olive oil, balsamic vinegar, salt, and pepper.
3. Drizzle the dressing over the tuna mixture and toss until well combined.
4. Serve with whole wheat pita bread on the side.

Day 15: Lentil Bolognese with Spaghetti Squash Noodles

Ingredients:

- 1 medium spaghetti squash
- 1 cup dry lentils, rinsed
- 1 onion, diced
- 2 carrots, grated
- 2 cloves garlic, minced
- 1 can (14 oz) crushed tomatoes
- 1 teaspoon dried oregano

- 1 teaspoon dried basil
- Salt and pepper to taste

Instructions:

1. Preheat the oven to 400°F (200°C).
2. Cut the spaghetti squash in half and remove the seeds. Place it on a baking sheet, cut side down.
3. Bake for 40-45 minutes or until the squash is tender. Scrape the flesh into "noodles."
4. In a pot, sauté onion, carrots, and garlic until softened.
5. Add lentils, crushed tomatoes, oregano, basil, salt, and pepper. Simmer until lentils are cooked.
6. Serve lentil Bolognese over spaghetti squash noodles.

Day 16: Baked Salmon with Lemon Dill Sauce and Quinoa Pilaf

Ingredients:

- 2 salmon fillets
- 1 cup quinoa, cooked
- 1/4 cup fresh dill, chopped
- 1 lemon, juiced and zested
- 2 tablespoons olive oil
- Salt and pepper to taste

Instructions:

1. Preheat the oven to 375°F (190°C).

2. Place salmon fillets on a baking sheet. Drizzle with olive oil, lemon juice, and zest. Sprinkle with chopped dill, salt, and pepper.
3. Bake for 15-20 minutes or until the salmon is cooked through.
4. Serve over a bed of cooked quinoa.

Day 17: Chicken Curry Stir-Fry with Bell Peppers and Brown Rice

Ingredients:

- 2 boneless, skinless chicken breasts, thinly sliced
- 2 bell peppers, sliced
- 1 onion, sliced
- 2 tablespoons curry powder
- 1 can (14 oz) coconut milk
- 1 tablespoon soy sauce
- 2 tablespoons olive oil
- Cooked brown rice

Instructions:

1. In a wok or large pan, heat olive oil. Stir-fry chicken until browned.
2. Add bell peppers and onion. Continue to stir-fry until vegetables are tender.
3. Sprinkle curry powder over the chicken and vegetables, stirring to coat.
4. Pour in coconut milk and soy sauce. Simmer until the sauce thickens.
5. Serve over cooked brown rice.

Day 18: Roasted Cauliflower Soup with Turmeric and Coconut Milk

Ingredients:

- 1 head cauliflower, chopped
- 1 onion, diced
- 2 cloves garlic, minced
- 1 teaspoon turmeric
- 4 cups vegetable broth
- 1 can (14 oz) coconut milk
- Salt and pepper to taste

Instructions:

1. Preheat the oven to 400°F (200°C).
2. Toss cauliflower, onion, and garlic with olive oil. Roast in the oven until cauliflower is golden.
3. Transfer roasted vegetables to a pot. Add turmeric, vegetable broth, and coconut milk.
4. Simmer for 15-20 minutes. Blend until smooth.
5. Season with salt and pepper before serving.

Day 19: Black Bean and Corn Salad with Avocado and Cilantro Lime Dressing

Ingredients:

- 2 cans (15 oz each) black beans, drained and rinsed
- 1 cup corn kernels (fresh or frozen)
- 1 avocado, diced

- 1/4 cup red onion, finely chopped
- 1/4 cup fresh cilantro, chopped
- Juice of 2 limes
- 2 tablespoons olive oil
- Salt and pepper to taste

Instructions:

1. In a large bowl, combine black beans, corn, avocado, red onion, and cilantro.
2. In a small bowl, whisk together lime juice, olive oil, salt, and pepper.
3. Pour the dressing over the salad and toss until well combined.

Day 20: Chicken Shawarma Bowl with Hummus, Tabouli, and Tahini Drizzle

Ingredients:

- 2 boneless, skinless chicken breasts, thinly sliced
- 1 tablespoon olive oil
- 1 tablespoon shawarma spice blend
- Hummus for serving
- Tabouli for serving
- Tahini sauce for drizzling

Instructions:

1. In a pan, heat olive oil. Cook chicken slices with shawarma spice blend until browned.
2. Assemble bowls with cooked chicken, hummus, tabouli, and a drizzle of tahini sauce.

Week 3: Ignite Your Energy

Day 21: Matcha Chia Seed Pudding with Berries and Almonds

Ingredients:

-   1 cup almond milk
-   2 tablespoons chia seeds
-   1 teaspoon matcha powder
-   1 tablespoon maple syrup
-   Mixed berries for topping
-   Sliced almonds for topping

- Instructions:

1. In a jar, whisk together almond milk, chia seeds, matcha powder, and maple syrup.
2. Refrigerate overnight or until the pudding thickens.
3. Top with mixed berries and sliced almonds before serving.

Day 22: Scrambled Eggs with Smoked Salmon and Asparagus

- Ingredients:

-   4 eggs

- 1/4 cup milk
- 4 oz smoked salmon
- 1/2 bunch asparagus, trimmed and chopped
- Salt and pepper to taste
- Chives for garnish

Instructions:

1. In a bowl, whisk together eggs and milk.
2. Scramble the eggs in a pan over medium heat.
3. Add smoked salmon and asparagus. Continue cooking until the asparagus is tender.
4. Season with salt and pepper. Garnish with chives.

Day 23: Spicy Shrimp Tacos with Mango Salsa and Avocado Crema

Ingredients:

- 1 lb shrimp, peeled and deveined
- 1 tablespoon olive oil
- 1 teaspoon chili powder
- 1/2 teaspoon cumin
- 1/2 teaspoon paprika
- 1/4 teaspoon cayenne pepper
- 1 cup mango, diced
- 1/4 cup red onion, finely chopped
- 1/4 cup cilantro, chopped
- Corn tortillas
- Avocado crema (blend avocado with lime juice and salt)

Instructions:

1. In a pan, heat olive oil. Toss shrimp with chili powder, cumin, paprika, and cayenne pepper. Cook until shrimp are pink.
2. In a bowl, mix mango, red onion, and cilantro to make salsa.
3. Assemble tacos with spicy shrimp, mango salsa, and a drizzle of avocado crema.

Day 24: Tofu Scramble with Turmeric and Roasted Vegetables

Ingredients:

- 1 block extra-firm tofu, crumbled
- 1 tablespoon olive oil
- 1/2 teaspoon turmeric
- 1/2 teaspoon cumin
- 1/4 teaspoon smoked paprika
- Salt and pepper to taste
- Mixed roasted vegetables (bell peppers, zucchini, cherry tomatoes)

Instructions:

1. In a pan, heat olive oil. Add crumbled tofu and cook until heated through.
2. Sprinkle turmeric, cumin, smoked paprika, salt, and pepper over the tofu. Stir to combine.
3. Serve with mixed roasted vegetables.

Day 25: Quinoa Buddha Bowl with Edamame, Roasted Sweet Potato, and Kimchi

Ingredients:

- 1 cup quinoa, cooked
- 1 cup edamame, shelled
- 1 sweet potato, cubed and roasted
- Kimchi
- Sesame seeds for garnish
- Soy sauce or tamari for drizzling

Instructions:

1. Assemble a bowl with cooked quinoa, edamame, roasted sweet potato, and kimchi.
2. Garnish with sesame seeds and drizzle with soy sauce or tamari.

Day 26: Grilled Chicken Breast with Chimichurri Sauce and Quinoa Salad

Ingredients:

- 2 boneless, skinless chicken breasts
- 1 cup quinoa, cooked
- Chimichurri sauce (parsley, cilantro, garlic, olive oil, red wine vinegar)
- Mixed greens for salad

Instructions:

1. Grill chicken breasts until cooked through.

2. Prepare chimichurri sauce by blending parsley, cilantro, garlic, olive oil, and red wine vinegar.
3. Assemble a plate with grilled chicken, quinoa salad, and mixed greens. Drizzle chimichurri sauce over the chicken.

Day 27: Beef and Broccoli Stir-Fry with Ginger and Garlic

Ingredients:

- 1 lb beef sirloin, thinly sliced
- 2 cups broccoli florets
- 2 tablespoons soy sauce
- 1 tablespoon oyster sauce
- 1 tablespoon hoisin sauce
- 1 tablespoon sesame oil
- 1 tablespoon cornstarch
- 1 tablespoon ginger, minced
- 2 cloves garlic, minced

Instructions:

1. In a bowl, mix beef slices with soy sauce, oyster sauce, hoisin sauce, sesame oil, and cornstarch.
2. Stir-fry marinated beef in a pan until browned. Remove from the pan.
3. In the same pan, stir-fry broccoli, ginger, and garlic until the broccoli is tender.
4. Add the cooked beef back to the pan. Toss until everything is coated and heated through.

Day 28: Lentil and Vegetable Soup with Fresh Herbs and Toasted Croutons

Ingredients:

- 1 cup dried lentils, rinsed
- 1 onion, diced
- 2 carrots, chopped
- 2 celery stalks, chopped
- 3 cloves garlic, minced
- 4 cups vegetable broth
- Fresh herbs (parsley, thyme, rosemary)
- Whole grain bread, cubed and toasted for croutons

Instructions:

1. In a large pot, sauté onion, carrots, celery, and garlic until softened.
2. Add lentils and vegetable broth. Bring to a boil, then simmer until lentils are tender.
3. Stir in fresh herbs. Serve with toasted whole grain croutons.

Day 29: Tropical Smoothie Bowl with Pineapple, Mango, and Coconut Milk

Ingredients:

- 1 cup frozen pineapple chunks
- 1/2 cup frozen mango chunks
- 1 banana

- 1/2 cup coconut milk
- Toppings: shredded coconut, chia seeds, granola, sliced banana

Instructions:

1. In a blender, blend pineapple, mango, banana, and coconut milk until smooth.
2. Pour into a bowl and top with shredded coconut, chia seeds, granola, and sliced banana.

Day 30: Grilled Salmon with Lemon Pepper Marinade and Roasted Root Vegetables

Ingredients:

- 2 salmon fillets
- 2 tablespoons olive oil
- Zest and juice of 1 lemon
- 1 teaspoon black pepper
- 1 teaspoon dried oregano
- 1 teaspoon paprika
- Mixed root vegetables (carrots, sweet potatoes, parsnips), chopped

Instructions:

1. Preheat the oven to 400°F (200°C).
2. In a bowl, mix olive oil, lemon zest, lemon juice, black pepper, oregano, and paprika.
3. Marinate salmon fillets in the mixture for at least 15 minutes.

4. Place marinated salmon on a baking sheet. Roast in the oven for 15-20 minutes.
5. Toss chopped root vegetables with olive oil, salt, and pepper. Roast alongside the salmon until vegetables are tender.
6. Serve grilled salmon over roasted root vegetables.

Recipe Index

Welcome to the comprehensive Recipe Index tailored for those seeking a vibrant and health-conscious culinary experience. Explore the following categories to discover delectable recipes designed to combat the four horsemen of aging: Oxidative Damage, Inflammation, Glycation, and Stress.

Grocery Shopping Guide

Elevate your shopping experience with this handy guide to ensure you have the freshest and healthiest ingredients on hand:

1. **Produce Section:**

   - Berries (for antioxidants)

   - Leafy greens (spinach, kale)

   - Colorful vegetables (tomatoes, bell peppers, sweet potatoes)

   - Fresh herbs (parsley, mint, cilantro)

2. **Protein Aisle:**

   - Salmon fillets (rich in omega-3 fatty acids)

   - Lean chicken breasts

   - Tofu (for anti-inflammatory and stress-relief recipes)

3. **Dry Goods and Grains:**

- Quinoa (for inflammation and glycation recipes)
- Chia seeds (for glycation and oxidative damage recipes)
- Whole wheat flour (for healthy baking)

4. **Spices and Herbs:**

- Turmeric (anti-inflammatory)
- Garlic (anti-inflammatory)
- Cumin, paprika, and curry spices (for anti-inflammatory recipes)
- Dried lavender (stress relief)

5. **Dairy and Alternatives:**

- Greek yogurt (for antioxidant smoothies)
- Feta cheese (for Mediterranean salads)
- Almond milk and coconut milk

6. **Sweeteners:**

- Honey (for natural sweetening)
- Dark chocolate (for stress-relief recipes)

Meal Prep Tips & Time-Saving Strategies

Efficiency meets culinary excellence with these meal prep tips and time-saving strategies:

1. **Batch Cooking:**

   - Prepare larger quantities and portion meals for the week.

   - Freeze individual servings for quick and convenient future use.

2. **Pre-Chop and Wash:**

   - Spend time prepping fruits and vegetables in advance for easy access during the week.

   - Wash and store leafy greens to streamline salad preparation.

3. **Strategic Ingredient Use:**

   - Choose versatile ingredients that can be used in multiple recipes.

   - Repurpose leftovers creatively to minimize waste.

4. **Utilize Appliances:**

   - Invest in time-saving kitchen appliances like a food processor or blender for quick meal preparation.

   - Use slow cookers or instant pots for hands-off cooking.

5. **Weekly Menu Planning:**

   - Plan your meals for the week to streamline grocery shopping.

- Rotate recipes to maintain a diverse and balanced diet.

Resources for Further Exploration

Delve deeper into the world of culinary wellness with additional resources:

1. **Nutrition Websites:**

   - Explore reputable nutrition websites for the latest information on anti-aging foods and dietary tips.

2. **Cookbooks and Blogs:**

   - Discover cookbooks and blogs dedicated to healthy aging recipes and lifestyle.

3. **Cooking Classes:**

   - Join online or local cooking classes focusing on anti-aging cuisines.

4. **Wellness Communities:**

   - Engage with online communities or forums to share experiences and gain insights into anti-aging nutrition.

5. **Books on Mindfulness and Stress Relief:**

   - Read books that explore the connection between mindfulness, stress relief, and overall well-being.

Embrace this Recipe Index as a gateway to not just recipes but a holistic approach to culinary well-being. Enhance your kitchen skills, save time, and continue your exploration of health-conscious living with the provided resources. Happy cooking and savoring the flavors of a vibrant life!